THE BROCKHAMPTON

book of
Herbal
Remedies

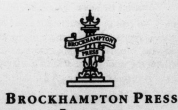

BROCKHAMPTON PRESS
LONDON

Contents

History of the Use of Herbal Remedies

The medicinal use of herbs is said to be as old as mankind itself. In early civilizations, food and medicine were linked, and many plants were eaten for their health-giving properties. In ancient Egypt, the slave workers were given a daily ration of garlic to help fight off the many fevers and infections that were common at that time. The first written records of herbs and their beneficial properties were compiled by the ancient Egyptians. Most of our knowledge and use of herbs can be traced back to the Egyptian priests who also practised herbal medicine. Records dating back to 1500 BC listed medicinal herbs, including caraway and cinnamon.

The ancient Greeks and Romans also carried out herbal medicine, and as they invaded new lands their doctors encountered new herbs and introduced herbs such as rosemary or lavender into new areas. Other cultures with a history of herbal medicine are the Chinese and the Indians. In Britain, the use of herbs rose and developed along with the establishment of monasteries around the country, each of which had its own herb garden for use in treating both the monks and the local people. In some areas, particularly Wales and Scotland, Druids and other Celtic healers are thought to have had an oral tradition of herbalism, where medicine was mixed with religion and ritual.

Over time, these healers and their knowledge led to the writing of the first 'herbals', which rapidly rose in importance and distribution upon the advent of the printing press in the 15th century. John Parkinson of London wrote a herbal around 1630, listing useful plants. Many herbalists set up their own apothecary shops, including the famous Nicholas Culpepper (1616–1654) whose most well-known work was *The Complete Herbal and English Physician, Enlarged* of 1649. Then in 1812, Henry Potter started a business supplying herbs and dealing in leeches. By this time a huge amount of traditional knowledge and folklore on medicinal herbs was available from Britain, Europe, the Middle East, Asia and the Americas. This promoted Potter to write *Potter's Encyclopaedia of Botanical Drugs and Preparations*, which is still published today.

It was in this period that scientifically inspired conventional medicine rose in popularity, sending herbal medicine into a decline. In rural areas, herbal medicine continued to thrive in local folklore, traditions and practices. 1864 brought about the foundation of the National Association (later Institute) of Medical Herbalists to organize training of herbal medicine practitioners and to maintain standards of practice. From 1864 until the early part of this century, the Institute fought attempts to ban herbal medicine and over time public interest in herbal medicine has increased, particularly over the last twenty years. This move away from synthetic drugs is partly due to possible side effects, bad publicity and public mistrust of the medical and pharmacological industries. The more natural appearance of herbal remedies has led to its growing support and popularity. Herbs from America have been incorporated with common remedies, and scientific research into herbs and their active ingredients has confirmed the healing power of herbs and enlarged the range of medicinal herbs used today.

Herbal medicine can be viewed as the precursor of modern pharmacology, but today it continues as an effective and more natural method of treating and preventing illness. Herbal medicine is three to four times more commonly practised than conventional medicine, worldwide.

Please note that this work is not intended to be comprehensive, and no one involved with the preparation or publication of this book can be held liable for any omissions, errors or for any consequences resulting from the use of this book.

Forms of Herbal Preparations

capsule: this is a gelatine container for swallowing and holding oils or balsams that would otherwise be difficult to administer due to their unpleasant taste or smell. It is used for cod liver oil or castor oil.

decoction: this is prepared using cut, bruised or ground bark and roots placed into a stainless steel or enamel pan (not aluminium) with cold water poured on. The mixture is boiled for 20–30 minutes, cooled and strained. It is best drunk when warm.

herbal dressing: this may be a compress or poultice. A compress is made of cloth or cotton wool soaked in cold or warm herbal decoctions or infusions while a poultice can be made with fresh or dried herbs. Bruised fresh herbs are applied directly to the affected area and dried herbs are made into a paste with water and placed on gauze on the required area. Both dressings are very effective in easing pain, swelling and inflammation of the skin and tissues.

infusion: this liquid is made from ground or bruised roots, bark, herbs or seeds by pouring boiling water onto the herb and leaving it to stand for 10–30 minutes, possibly stirring the mixture occasionally. The resultant liquid is strained and used. Cold infusions may be made if the active principles are yielded from the herb without heat. Today, infusions may be packaged into teabags for convenience.

liquid extract: this preparation, if correctly made, is the most concentrated fluid form in which herbal drugs may be obtained and, as such, is very popular and convenient. Each herb is treated by various means depending on the individual properties of the herb, e.g. cold percolation, high pressure, evaporation by heat in a vacuum. These extracts are commonly held in a household stock of domestic remedies.

pessary: similar to suppositories, but it is used in female complaints to apply drugs to the walls of the vagina and cervix.

pill: probably the best known and most widely used herbal preparation. It is normally composed of concentrated extracts and alkaloids, in combination with active crude drugs. The pill may be coated with sugar or another pleasant-tasting substance that is readily soluble in the stomach.

solid extract: this type of preparation is prepared by evaporating the fresh juices or strong infusions of herbal drugs to the consistency of honey. It may also be prepared from an alcoholic tincture base. This preparation is used mainly to produce pills, plasters, ointments and compressed tablets.

suppository: this preparation is a small cone of a convenient and easily soluble base with herbal extracts added, which are used to apply medicines to the rectum. It is very effective in treatment of piles, cancers etc.

tablet: this is made by compressing drugs into a small compass. It is more easily administered and has a quicker action as it dissolves more rapidly in the stomach.

tincture: this is the most prescribed form of herbal medicine. It is based on alcohol and, as such, removes certain active principles from herbs that will not dissolve in water, or in the presence of heat. The tincture produced is long-lasting, highly concentrated and only needs to be taken in small doses for beneficial effects. The ground or chopped dried herb is placed in a container with 40 per cent alcohol such as gin or vodka and left for two weeks. The tincture is then decanted into a dark bottle and sealed before use.

aconite   *Aconitum napellus*

Common name: monkshood, blue rocket, friar's cap, wolfsbane.
Occurrence: indigenous to mountain slopes in the Alps and
Pyrenees. Introduced into England very early, before 900 AD.
Parts used: the leaves used fresh and the root when dried. It
contains alkaloidal material—aconitine, benzaconine and
aconine among other compounds.
Medicinal uses: the plant is poisonous and should not be
used except under medical advice. It is an anodyne,
diaphoretic, febrifuge and sedative. Used for reducing fever
and inflammation in the treatment of catarrh, tonsillitis and
croup. It may be used in controlling heart spasm.
Administered as: tincture, liniment and occasionally as
hypodermic injection.

alder   *Alnus glutinosa*

Common name: Betula alnus
Occurrence: commonly found throughout Britain, usually in
moist woods or by streams.
Parts used: bark and leaves. The bark, wood, shoots, catkins
and leaves have all been used as dyes. The bark and leaves
contain tannic acid.
Medicinal uses: tonic and astringent. Used as a decoction to
bathe swelling and inflammation, particularly of the throat.
Administered as: decoction.

aloes   *Alde perryi, Alde vera*

Occurrence: indigenous to East and South Africa and
introduced into the West Indies.
Parts used: the drug, aloes, is described as "the liquid
evaporated to dryness that drains from the leaves." It
contains two aloin compounds, barbaloin and isobarbaldin,
as well as amorphous aloin, resin and aloe-emodin in
differing proportions.
Medicinal uses: emmenagogue, purgative, vermifuge, anthel-

9

mintic. It is generally administered along with carminative and anodyne drugs, and acts on the lower bowel. The liquid form may be used externally to ease skin irritation.
Administered as: fluid extract, powdered extract, decoction, tincture.

anemone pulsatilla   *Anemone pulsatilla*
Common name: pasque flower, meadow anemone, wind flower
Occurrence: found locally in chalk downs and limestone areas of England.
Parts used: the whole herb. It produces oil of anemone upon distillation with water.
Medicinal uses: nervine, antispasmodic, alterative and diaphoretic. It is beneficial in disorders of mucous membranes and of the respiratory and digestive passages. Can be used to treat asthma, whooping cough and bronchitis and used as a homoeopathic remedy.
Administered as: fluid extract.

arnica   *Arnica montana*
Common name: mountain tobacco, leopard's bane
Occurrence: indigenous to central Europe but found in England and southern Scotland.
Parts used: rhizome and flowers. They contain arnicin, tannin, phullin and a volatile oil.
Medicinal uses: stimulant, vulnerary and diuretic. It is used in external application to bruises and sprains but is rarely used internally as it irritates the stomach, and may cause severe poisoning. A tincture has been used to treat epilepsy and seasickness.
Administered as: tincture, lotion, poultice.

asparagus   *Asparagus officinalis*
Common name: sparrow grass.

Occurrence: a rare native in Britain but found wild on the southwest coast of England.
Parts used: root.
Medicinal uses: this plant has diuretic, laxative, cardiac and sedative effects. It is recommended in cases of dropsy.
Administered as: expressed juice, decoction or made in a syrup.

avens *Geum urbanum*
Common name: colewort, herb Bennet, city avens, wild rue, way Bennet, goldy star, clove root.
Occurrence: a common hedgerow plant in Great Britain and Europe.
Parts used: herb and root. The herb contains a volatile oil composed of eugenol and a glucoside, while the root also contains tannin.
Medicinal uses: it is an astringent, styptic, febrifuge, sudorific, stomachic, antiseptic, tonic and aromatic. It is useful in diarrhoea, sore throat, chills, fevers and headache amongst other complaints. An infusion may be used for skin problems, as a wash.
Administered as: an infusion, decoction or tincture.

balm *Melissa officinalis*
Common name: sweet balm, lemon balm, honey plant, cure-all.
Occurrence: a common garden plant in Great Britain naturalized into southern England at a very early period.
Parts used: the herb.
Medicinal uses: as a carminative, diaphoretic, or febrifuge. It can be made into a cooling tea for fever patients and balm is often used in combination with other herbs to treat colds and fever.
Administered as: an infusion.

basil   *Ocimum basilicum*

Common name: sweet basil, garden basil.
Occurrence: as a garden plant throughout Britain.
Parts used: the herb. It contains an aromatic, volatile, camphoraceous oil.
Medicinal uses: aromatic with carminative and cooling properties. It is used to treat mild nervous disorders and an infusion of basil is said to be good for obstructions of the internal organs and in stopping vomiting and nausea.
Administered as: a flavouring in food, dried leaves or an infusion.

belladonna   *Atropa belladonna*

Common name: deadly nightshade, devil's cherries, dwale, black cherry, devil's herb, great morel.
Occurrence: native to central and southern Europe but commonly grows in England.
Parts used: roots and leaves. The root contains several alkaloid compounds including hyoscyamine, atropine and belladonnine. The same alkaloids are present in the leaves but the amount of each compound varies according to plant type and methods of storing and drying leaves.
Medicinal uses: as a narcotic, diuretic, sedative, mydriatic, antispasmodic. The drug is used as an anodyne in febrile conditions, night sweats and coughs. It is valuable in treating eye diseases and is used as a pain-relieving lotion to treat neuralgia, gout, rheumatism and sciatica. Belladonna is an extremely poisonous plant and should always be used under medical supervision. Cases of accidental poisoning and death are well known. Despite this, it is a valuable drug used to treat a wide range of disease.
Administered as: a liquid extract that is used to produce alcoholic extracts, plasters, liniment, suppositories, tincture and ointment.

birch, common
Betula alba

Common name: white birch, bouleau, berke, bereza.

Occurrence: common in Europe, from Sicily to Iceland, and also found in northern Asia.

Parts used: bark and leaves. The bark contains tannic acid, behilin and behils camphor while the leaves contain betulorentic acid.

Medicinal uses: it is bitter and astringent. The bark yields oil of birch tar upon destructive distillation, which is similar to oil of wintergreen. The oil is used in skin disease ointments, e.g. treating eczema, and is also a component of insect repellent. Birch tea made of the leaves is recommended for gout, rheumatism and dropsy and is also said to be good for breaking up kidney stones. Sap from the tree is used to produce beer, wine, spirits and vinegar in parts of Europe.

Administered as: oil, infusion.

birthwort
Aristolochia longa

Common name: long-rooted birthwort.

Occurrence: throughout Europe and Great Britain.

Parts used: the root, which contains aristolochine.

Medicinal uses: aromatic and stimulant. It is useful in treating gout and rheumatism and may be used to clear obstructions after childbirth.

Administered as: powdered root.

bittersweet
Solanum dulcamara

Common name: woody nightshade, violet bloom, scarlet berry, felonwood, felonwort, dulcamara.

Occurrence: a climbing plant found in hedgerows through-out Britain.

Parts used: twigs and root bark. The twigs contain the alkaloid solamine and the glucoside dulcamarine, which gives bittersweet its characteristic taste. It also contains sugar, gum, starch and resin.

Medicinal uses: narcotic, resolvent, diuretic and alterative. It promotes all secretions, particularly of the skin and kidneys, and is generally used to clear stubborn skin eruptions, scrofula and ulcers, and has been recommended in chronic bronchial catarrh, asthma or whooping cough. In large doses, the drug can cause paralysis of the central nervous system and lead to death.
Administered as: a fluid extract, decoction.

blackberry   *Rubus fructicosus*
Common name: bramble, bumble-kite, bramble-kite, bly, brummel, brameberry, scaldhead, brambleberry.
Occurrence: common throughout Britain.
Parts used: root and leaves, which both contain tannin.
Medicinal uses: as astringent and tonic. It is valuable against dysentery and diarrhoea. A decoction of the root was used to treat whooping cough. A cordial or vinegar drink was made and is useful in treating looseness of the bowels, piles or a feverish cold.
Administered as: decoction, fluid extract or made into cordial, wine or vinegar.

blackcurrant   *Ribes nigrum*
Common name: quinsy berries, squinancy berries.
Occurrence: a common garden plant in Britain but truly native only to Yorkshire and the Lake District; also found in Europe.
Parts used: fruit, leaves, bark and root.
Medicinal uses: diuretic, diaphoretic, febrifuge, refrigerant, detergent. The fruit juice is excellent in febrile diseases and as an extract is good for sore throats. The infused leaves are cleansing while a root infusion is used in eruptive fevers and has been used to treat cattle. A decoction of the bark is effective against calculus, oedema and haemorrhoids. The fruit was commonly used to make jelly, wine and cheese.
Administered as: juice, infusion or decoction.

blue flag *Iris versicolor*

Common name: poison flag, flag lily, liver lily, snake lily, dragon flower, dagger flower, water flag.

Occurrence: indigenous to North America and introduced into Britain and Europe and now a common garden plant.

Parts used: the rhizome, which contains starch, gum, tannin, isophthalic acid, salicylic acid and oleoresin of which the latter compound contains the medicinal properties.

Medicinal uses: alterative, diuretic, cathartic, stimulant. It is chiefly used for its alterative properties being useful as a purgative in disorders of the liver and the duodenum. Also, combined with other herbs as a blood purifier, or used alone against syphilis, scrofula, skin afflictions and dropsy.

Administered as: powdered root, solid extract, fluid extract or tincture.

bogbean *Menyanthes trifoliata*

Common name: buckbean, marsh trefoil, water trefoil, marsh clover, boonan.

Occurrence: in spongy bogs, marshes and shallow water throughout Europe and is more common in northern England and Scotland.

Parts used: the herb, which consists of volatile oil and a glucoside called menyanthin.

Medicinal uses: as a tonic, cathartic, deobstruent and febrifuge. A liquid extract is used to treat rheumatism, scurvy and skin complaints. It has also been used as an external application to reduce glandular swelling. In the Scottish Highlands it was used to remedy stomach pains caused by ulcers and was also brewed into beer and smoked as herb tobacco. It is thought to cure ague (malaria) where other cures have failed.

Administered as: the liquid extract, infusion or as tea.

boneset *Eupatonium perfoliatum*

Common name: thoroughwort, Indian sage, feverwort.

Occurrence: found in meadows and damp ground in North America and Europe.

Parts used: the herb. The important constituents are volatile oil, tannic acid, gum, resin, sugar and the glucoside eupatonin.

Medicinal uses: a diaphoretic, tonic, febrifuge, expectorant, stimulant and laxative. It is used to treat rheumatism, colds and influenza, catarrh and skin diseases. It acts slowly on the stomach, liver, bowel and uterus but has a persistent beneficial effect. In large doses it is an emetic and purgative.

Administered as: powdered herb, fluid extract and solid extract.

broom   *Cytisus scoparius*

Common name: broom tops, Irish tops, basam, bizzom, browne, brum, bream, green broom.

Occurrence: indigenous to England and commonly found on heathland throughout Britain, Europe and northern Asia.

Parts used: the young herbaceous tops, which contain sparteine and scoparin as the active components.

Medicinal uses: diuretic and cathartic. The broom tops may be used as a decoction or infusion to aid dropsy while if the tops are pressed and treated broom juice is obtained. This fluid extract is generally used in combination with other diuretic compounds. An infusion of broom, agrimony and DANDELION root is excellent in remedying bladder, kidney and liver trouble. *Cytisus* should be used carefully as the sparteine has a strong effect on the heart and, depending upon dose, can cause weakness of the heart similar to that caused by HEMLOCK (*Conium maculatum*). Death can occur in extreme cases if the respiratory organ's activity is impaired.

Administered as: fluid extract and infusion.

bryony, white   *Bryonica dioica, Bryonica alba*

Common name: English mandrake, wild vine, wild hops, lady's seal, tetterbury, wild nep, tamus.

Occurrence: a native of Europe, frequently found in England but rare in Scotland.
Parts used: the root.
Medicinal uses: irritative, hydrogogue, cathartic. It was previously used as a purgative drug but these and other uses have been discontinued on account of its highly irritant nature. It is still used in small doses for coughs, influenza, bronchitis and pneumonia. It is useful in cardiac disorders caused by gout or rheumatism and in malarial and contagious diseases. Care should be taken when used, due to its poisonous nature.
Administered as: liquid extract.

burdock
Artium lappa

Common name: lappa, fox's clote, thorny burr, beggar's buttons, cockle buttons, love leaves, philanthropium, personata, happy major, clot-bur.
Occurrence: freely found in ditches and hedgerows throughout England and Europe but rare in Scotland.
Parts used: root, herb and seeds (fruits). They contain the chemicals inulin, mucilage, sugar and tannic acid along with a crystalline glucoside, lappin.
Medicinal uses: alterative, diuretic and diaphoretic. It is an excellent blood purifier and effective in remedying all skin diseases. The root is most powerful and has anti-scorbutic properties that make it very useful for boils, scurvy and rheumatism. Also used as a wash for ulcers, a poultice for tumours, gouty swellings and bruises. An infusion of the leaves aids the stomach and eases indigestion. The tincture obtained from the seeds is a relaxant, demulcent and skin tonic.
Administered as: a fluid extract, infusion, tincture and solid extract.

burr marigold
Bidens impartica

Common name: water agrimony.

Occurrence: commonly found in wet places in England but less frequently seen in Scotland.
Parts used: the whole plant.
Medicinal uses: astringent, diaphoretic, diuretic. This plant has been useful in dropsy, gout, haematuria and fevers. It is very good in treating diseases of the respiratory organs where bleeding occurs and also in uterine haemorrhage.
Administered as: an infusion.

butterbur *Petasites vulgaris*

Common name: langwort, umbrella plant, bog rhubarb, plapperdock, blatterdock, capdockin, bogshorns, butterdock.
Occurrence: in low wet grounds, marshy meadows and riversides in Great Britain.
Parts used: rhizome or root stock.
Medicinal uses: as a cardiac tonic, stimulant, and diuretic. It is good as a remedy for fevers, asthma, colds, urinary complaints, gravel and plague. It is also taken as a homoeopathic remedy for severe neuralgia in the back and loins. Recently, the use of butterbur has been recommended in easing the pain of migraine and painful menstruation. One of the most important developments is the treatment of cancer with *Petasites* where the drug attacks tumours and abnormal cell changes very strongly and, in clinical tests, it has been shown to slow or stop the cancer spreading through the body. It has also become an effective remedy for severe asthma.
Administered as: a decoction and tincture.

camomile *Anthemis nobilis*

Common name: Roman camomile, double camomile, manzanilla (Spanish), maythen (Saxon).
Occurrence: low-growing plant found wild in the British Isles.
Parts used: flowers and herb. The active principles therein are

a volatile oil, anthemic acid, tannic acid and a glucoside.
Medicinal uses: tonic, stomachic, anodyne and anti-spasmodic.
An infusion of camomile tea is a very effective remedy for
hysterical and nervous afflictions in women, as well as an
emmenagogue. It has a powerful soothing and sedative
effect that is harmless. A tincture is used to cure diarrhoea
in children, and it is used with purgatives to prevent griping,
and as a tonic it helps dropsy. Externally, it can be applied
alone or with other herbs as a poultice to relieve pain,
swellings, inflammation and neuralgia. Its strong antiseptic
properties make it invaluable for reducing swelling of the
face due to abscess or injury. As a lotion, the flowers are
good for resolving toothache and earache. The herb itself is
an ingredient in herb beers. The use of camomile can be
dated back to ancient Egyptian times when it was dedicated
to the sun because of its extensive healing properties.
Administered as: decoction, infusion, fluid extract and
essential oil.

caraway   *Carum carvi*
Common name: caraway seed, caraway fruit, alcaravea.
Occurrence: common in Europe and Asia, naturalized in
Britain.
Parts used: the fruit, which produces a volatile oil containing a hydrocarbon, carvene, and an oxygenated oil, carvol.
Medicinal uses: aromatic, stimulant and carminative. It was
widely used as a cordial to ease dyspepsia and hysteria. The
oil is applied to treat flatulence and stomach disorders.
Distilled caraway water is used to ease flatulent colic in
infants and is an excellent children's medicine. The bruised
fruits were used to remove pain from bad earache and was
also used as a poultice to take away bruises. Caraway is
widely used as a flavouring for cheeses and seed-cakes.
Administered as: a liquid extract and poultice.

catmint   *Nepeta cataria*
Common name: catnep, nep.
Occurrence: a wild English plant found in hedges, field
borders and waste ground; found localized in Scotland.
Parts used: the herb.
Medicinal uses: carminative, tonic, diaphoretic, refrigerant,
mildly stimulating and slightly emmenagogue. This herb is
good in treating colds, fevers, restlessness and colic. It is
also used in nervousness and insanity and to calm children
and soothe nightmares when taken as an infusion or conserve.
It can be applied to swellings and bruises as a poultice.
Administered as: an infusion, injection or poultice.

celandine   *Chelidonium majus*
Common name: garden celandine, common celandine,
greater celandine.
Occurrence: common in gardens, hedges and waste ground
in Great Britain and Europe.
Parts used: the herb, which contains the alkaloids chelidanine,
chelerythrin (the latter is narcotic), homochelidonine A and
B. Three other major chemicals are found in the plant.
Medicinal uses: alterative, diuretic and purgative. It is of
benefit to jaundice, eczema, scrofulous diseases and scurvy.
The fresh juice was used to cure warts, ringworm and corns
but should not otherwise be allowed to come into direct
contact with the skin. In various forms, it has previously
been effective against itching, piles, toothache and cancer.
Administered as: an infusion, fluid extract, decoction, lotion
and poultice.

celery   *Apium graveolens*
Common name: smallage, wild celery.
Occurrence: native to southern Europe; cultivated in Britain.
Parts used: the ripe seeds, herb and root of which the seeds
contain two oils and apiol.

Medicinal uses: carminative, stimulant, diuretic, tonic, nervine and aphrodisiac. It is utilized as a tonic in combination with other herbs, promoting restfulness, sleep and lack of hysteria and is excellent in relieving rheumatism.
Administered as: fluid extract, essential oil, powdered seeds.

chickweed   *Stellania media*
Common name: starweed, star chickweed, *Alsine media*, passerina.
Occurrence: native to all temperate and north Arctic regions and naturalized where humans have settled. A common weed.
Parts used: the whole herb, both fresh and dried.
Medicinal uses: demulcent, refrigerant. It is good as a poultice to reduce inflammation and heal indolent ulcers, but is most important as an ointment in treating eye problems and cutaneous diseases. It will also benefit scurvy and kidney disorders as an infusion.
Administered as: an infusion, poultice and ointment.

clover, red   *Trifolium pratense*
Common name: trefoil, purple clover.
Occurrence: widely distributed in Britain and Europe.
Parts used: flowers.
Medicinal uses: alterative, sedative, antispasmodic. The fluid extract or infusion are excellent in treating bronchial and whooping coughs. External applications of the herb in a poultice has been used on cancerous growths.
Administered as: fluid extract and infusion.

club moss   *Lycopodium clavatum*
Common name: lycopodium, lycopodium seed, vegetable sulphur, wolf's claw, muscus terrestris repens.
Occurrence: occurs throughout Great Britain, being most plentiful on heath or moorland in northern countries and also found all over the world.

Parts used: the fresh plant and spores.

Medicinal uses: spores are diuretic, nervine and aperient. The fresh plant has been used as a stomachic and a diuretic herb in calculus and kidney complaints. The spores are currently applied externally to wounds and taken internally for diarrhoea, dysentery, gout and scurvy.

Administered as: dried spores, fresh moss.

coltsfoot   *Tussilago farfara*

Common name: coughwort, hallfoot, horsehoof, ass's foot, foals-wort, fieldhove, bullsfoot, donnhove.

Occurrence: commonly found wild on waste ground and riverbanks in Great Britain.

Parts used: leaves, flowers and root.

Medicinal uses: demulcent, expectorant and tonic. Coltsfoot is one of the most popular cough remedies and is generally taken in conjunction with horehound, MARSHMALLOW or GROUND IVY. It has been called "nature's best herb for the lungs" and it was recommended that the leaves be smoked to relieve a cough. Today, it forms the basis of British herb tobacco along with BOGBEAN, EYEBRIGHT, wood betony, ROSEMARY, THYME, LAVENDER and CAMOMILE, WHICH is said to relieve asthma, catarrh, bronchitis and lung troubles.

Administered as: syrup or smoked when dried.

comfrey   *Symphytum officinale*

Common name: common comfrey, knitbone, knitback, bruise-wort, slippery root, gum plant, consolida, ass ear, blackwort.

Occurrence: a native of Europe and temperate Asia but common throughout England by rivers and ditches.

Parts used: root and leaves. The roots contain a large quantity of mucilage, choline and allantoin.

Medicinal uses: demulcent, mildly astringent, expectorant and vulnerary. It is frequently used in pulmonary complaints, to soothe intestinal trouble and is a gentle remedy for diarrhoea and dysentery. A strong decoction or tea is given in cases of internal haemorrhage, e.g. the lungs, stomach, bowels or haemorrhoids. Externally, the leaves have been used as a poultice to promote healing of severe cuts, ulcers and abscesses and to reduce swelling, sprains and bruises. Allantoin reduces swelling round damaged or fractured bones, thus allowing healing to occur faster and more thoroughly. *Administered as*: a decoction, poultice and liquid extract.

costmary *Tanacetum balsamita*
Common name: alecost, balsam herb, costmarie, mace, balsamita.
Occurrence: an old English herb naturalized from the Orient in the 16th century.
Parts used: leaves.
Medicinal uses: it was formerly used as an aperient, antiseptic and astringent herb in treating dysentery. Used as an infusion to heal stomach and head problems but also as flavouring for ale and in salads.
Administered as: infusion and tincture.

couchgrass *Agropyrum repens*
Common name: twitchgrass, Scotch quelch, quickgrass, dog's grass, *Triticum repens*.
Occurrence: abundant in fields and waste ground in Britain, Europe, northern Asia and North and South America.
Parts used: rhizome. It contains triticin (a carbohydrate).
Medicinal uses: diuretic, demulcent, aperient. Widely used in complaints of the urinary organs and bladder. Also recommended for gout and rheumatism.
Administered as: an infusion, decoction and liquid extract.

cowslip *Primula veris*
Common name: herb Peter, paigle, peggle, key flower, key of heaven, fairy cups, petty mulleins, patsywort, plumrocks, mayflower, Our Lady's keys, arthritica.

Occurrence: a common wild flower in all parts of Britain.
Parts used: the flower.
Medicinal uses: sedative, antispasmodic. It is very good in relieving restlessness and insomnia. Commonly brewed into a wine that was a good children's medicine in small doses.
Administered as: an infusion or wine.

cucumber   *Cucumis sativa*
Common name: cowcumber.
Occurrence: a native of the East Indies but first cultivated in Britain around 1573.
Parts used: the whole fruit, peeled or unpeeled, raw or cooked.
Medicinal uses: the seeds are diuretic and are an excellent taeniacide and purge. The fruit is very good as a skin cosmetic as it has cooling, healing and soothing effects on irritated skin. Cucumber juice is widely utilized in emollient ointments or creams and is good for sunburn.
Administered as: expressed juice, lotion or ointment.

daffodil   *Narcissus pseudo-narcissus*
Common name: narcissus, porillion, daffy-down-dilly, fleur de coucou, Lent lily.
Occurrence: found wild in most European countries including the British Isles.
Parts used: the bulb, leaves and flowers. The bulbs contain an alkaloid called lyconine.
Medicinal uses: the flowers, when powdered, have emetic properties and as an infusion are used in pulmonary catarrh. The bulbs are also emetic and, indeed, can cause people to collapse and die due to paralysis of the central nervous system due to the action of lyconine, which acts quickly. Accidents have resulted from daffodil bulbs being mistaken for onions and eaten. Since high temperatures and cooking does not break down the poisonous alkaloid, considerable care should be taken to avoid problems. The bulbs are used

externally as an astringent poultice to dissolve hard swellings and aid wound healing.
Administered as: powder and extract.

daisy, common
Bellis perennis

Common name: bruisewort, bairnwort, eye of the day.
Occurrence: very common all over the British Isles.
Parts used: the root and leaves.
Medicinal uses: it was formerly utilized as a cure for fresh
wounds, pains and aches and was taken internally as
distilled water to treat fevers and inflammation of the liver.
Administered as: a poultice and distilled water.

daisy, ox-eye
Chrysanthemum leuconthemum

Common name: great ox-eye, goldens, marguerite, moon
daisy, horse gowan, maudlin daisy, field daisy, dun daisy,
butter daisy, horse daisy, maudlinwort, white weed, gowan.
Occurrence: found in fields in Europe and northern Asia.
Parts used: the whole herb, flowers and root.
Medicinal uses: antispasmodic, diuretic, tonic. This herb's
main use has been in whooping cough, asthma and nervous
excitability. When taken as a tonic, it acts in a similar way to
CAMOMILE flowers and calms night sweats and nightmares. An
infusion of ox-eye daisy flowers is good at relieving bronchial coughs and catarrh. It is also used as a lotion for
wounds, bruises and ulcers.
Administered as: an infusion and lotion.

dandelion
Taraxacum officinale

Common name: priest's crown, swine's snout.
Occurrence: widely found across the northern temperate
zone in pastures, meadows and waste ground.
Parts used: the root and leaves. The main constituents of the
root are taraxacin, a bitter substance, and taraxacerin, an
acid resin, along with the sugar inulin.

Medicinal uses: diuretic, tonic and slightly aperient. It acts as a general body stimulant, but chiefly acts on the liver and kidneys. Dandelion is used as a bitter tonic in atonic dyspepsia as a mild laxative and to promote increased appetite and digestion. The herb is best used in combination with other herbs and is used in many patent medicines. Roasted dandelion root is also used as a coffee substitute and helps ease dyspepsia, gout and rheumatism.

Administered as: fluid extract, decoction, infusion, tincture, solid extract and juice.

dill   *Peucedanum graveolus, Fructus anethi*

Common name: dill seed, dill fruit, *Anethum graveolus, Fructus anethi*.

Occurrence: indigenous to Mediterranean districts and south Russia and cultivated in England and Europe.

Parts used: the dried ripe fruit. An oil obtained from the fruit is almost identical to oil of caraway, both containing limonene and carvone.

Medicinal uses: stimulant, aromatic, carminative and stomachic. It is usually given as dillwater, which is very good for children's flatulence or disordered digestion. Oil of dill is used in medicine in largely the same way, but is also used in perfuming soaps.

Administered as: distilled water, essential oil.

dock, yellow   *Rumex crispus*

Common name: curled dock.

Occurrence: normally found on roadside ditches and waste ground all over Britain.

Parts used: the root and whole herb.

Medicinal uses: the root has laxative, alterative and a mildly tonic action and is used in rheumatism, bilious complaints and haemorrhoids. It is very useful in treating jaundice, diseases of the blood, scurvy, chronic skin diseases and as a

tonic on the digestive system. Yellow dock is said to have a positive effect on slowing the development of cancer, due to its alterative and tonic properties. It has similar effects to that of RHUBARB and has been used in treating diphtheria.
Administered as: dried extract, syrup, infusion, tincture, ointment, fluid extract and solid extract.

dog-rose
Rosa canina

Common name: wild briar, hip tree, cynosbatos.
Occurrence: indigenous to Britain.
Parts used: the ripe fruit, which contain invert fruit sugars, a range of mineral salts and a large proportion of vitamin C or ascorbic acid.
Medicinal uses: astringent, refrigerant and pectoral. The fruit is used in strengthening the stomach and digestion, as well as easing coughs. It is made into an uncooked preserve, a syrup that is excellent for infants and children and rose-hip tea has very beneficial effects. An infusion of dog-rose leaves has been used as a tea substitute and has a pleasant aroma.
Administered as: an infusion, syrup or dietary item.

elder
Sambucus nigra

Common name: black elder, common elder, European elder, pipe tree, bore tree, bour tree.
Occurrence: frequently seen in Europe and Britain.
Parts used: bark, leaves, flowers and berries.
Medicinal uses: the bark is a strong purgative and in large doses is emetic. It has been used successfully in epilepsy, and a tincture of the young bark relieves asthmatic symptoms and croup in children. A tea made from the roots was highly effective against dropsy. The leaves are used both fresh and dried and contain the alkaloid sambucine, a glucoside called sambunigrin, as well as hydrogenic acid, cane sugar and potassium nitrate among other compounds. The leaves are used in preparation of green elder ointment, which is used

domestically for bruises, haemorrhoids, sprains, chilblains and applied to wounds. Elder leaves have the same purgative effects as the bark (but produce more nausea) and have expectorant, diaphoretic and diuretic actions.

The elder flowers are either distilled into elderflower water or dried. The water is used in eye and skin lotions as it is mildly astringent and a gentle stimulant. When infused, the dried flowers make elderflower tea, which is gently laxative, aperient and diaphoretic. It is an old-fashioned remedy for colds and influenza when taken hot, before bed. The tea is also recommended to be drunk before breakfast as a blood purifier. Elder flowers would also be made into a lotion or poultice for use on inflamed areas and into an ointment that was good on wounds, scalds and burns. The ointment was used on the battlefields in World War I and at home for chapped hands and chilblains.

Administered as: an infusion, tincture, ointment, syrup, lotion, distilled water, poultice and dried powder.

elm, common   *Ulmus campestris*

Common name: field elm, ulmi cortex, broad-leaved elm.
Occurrence: common in Britain, Europe, Asia and North Africa.
Parts used: the dried inner bark.
Medicinal uses: tonic, demulcent, astringent and diuretic. It was formerly employed as an antiscorbutic decoction recommended in skin diseases such as ringworm. Also used as a poultice to relieve pain from gout or rheumatism.
Administered as: tincture, fluid extract or tea.

evening primrose   *Oenothera biennis*

Common name: tree primrose, sun drop.
Occurrence: native to North America but naturalized in British and European gardens.
Parts used: the bark and leaves.
Medicinal uses: astringent, sedative. The drug from this herb

is not extensively used but has been of benefit for gastro-intestinal disorders, dyspepsia, liver torpor and in female problems in association with pelvic illness. It has also been successfully used in whooping cough and spasmodic asthma.
Administered as: liquid extract.

eyebright   *Euphrasia officinalis*
Common name: euphrasia.
Occurrence: a wild plant growing in meadows and grasslands in England and Europe.
Parts used: the herb. This plant contains various chemicals including euphrasia-tannin, mannite and glucose.
Medicinal uses: slightly tonic and astringent. As its name suggests, eyebright is recommended in treating diseases of the sight, weak eyes etc. It is generally used as an infusion in water or milk and is combined in a lotion with golden seal, the pairing said to be highly effective.
Administered as: infusion, ointment or expressed juice.

fennel   *Foeniculum vulgare*
Common name: hinojo, fenkel, sweet fennel, wild fennel.
Occurrence: found wild in most areas of temperate Europe and generally considered indigenous to the Mediterranean; cultivated for medicinally in France, Russia, India and Persia.
Parts used: seeds, leaves and roots. The roots are rarely used in herbal medicine today. The essential oil is separated by distillation with water. Fennel oil varies widely in quality and composition dependent upon where and under what conditions the fennel was grown.
Medicinal uses: aromatic, stimulant, carminative and stomachic. The herb is principally used with purgatives to allay their tendency to griping, and the seeds form an ingredient of the compound liquorice powder. Fennel water also acts in a similar manner to dill water in correcting infant flatulence.
Administered as: fluid extract, distilled water, essential oil.

feverfew   *Chrysanthemum parthenium*

Common name: featherfew, featherfoil, flirtwort, bachelor's buttons, pyrethrum parthenium.

Occurrence: wild in hedgerows in many areas of Europe and Britain.

Parts used: the herb.

Medicinal uses: aperient, carminative, bitter, stimulant, emmenagogue. It is employed in hysterical complaints, nervousness and low spirits as a general tonic. A decoction is made and is useful in easing coughs, wheezing and difficult breathing. Earache was relieved by a cold infusion while a tincture of feverfew eased the pain and swelling caused after insect or vermin bites. The herb was planted around dwellings to purify the atmosphere and ward off disease.

Administered as: warm or cold infusion, poultice, tincture, decoction.

flax   *Linum usitatissimum*

Common name: linseed.

Occurrence: grows in most temperate and tropical countries.

Parts used: the seeds and oil expressed from the seeds, a cake remains that can be ground up to form linseed meal.

Medicinal uses: emollient, demulcent, pectoral. A poultice of linseed meal, either alone or with mustard, is effective in relieving pain and irritation from boils, ulcers, inflamed areas and abscesses. Flax is normally utilized as an addition to cough medicines, while linseed oil is sometimes given as a laxative or to remove gravel and stones. When mixed with lime water the oil is excellent on burns and scalds.

Administered as: essential oil, ground seed coats (meal), infusion, syrup and poultice.

foxglove   *Digitalis purpurea*

Common name: witch's gloves, dead men's bells, fairy's glove, gloves of Our Lady, bloody fingers, virgin's glove, fairy caps, folk's glove, fairy thimbles, fair women's plant.

Occurrence: indigenous and widely distributed throughout Great Britain and Europe.

Parts used: the leaves, which contain four important glucosides—digitoxin, digitalin, digitalein and digitonin—of which the first three listed are cardiac stimulants.

Medicinal uses: cardiac tonic, sedative, diuretic. Administering digitalis increases the activity of all forms of muscle tissue, particularly the heart and arterioles. It causes a very high rise in blood pressure and the pulse is slowed and becomes regular. Digitalis causes the heart to contract in size, allowing increased blood flow and nutrient delivery to the organ. It also acts on the kidneys and is a good remedy for dropsy, particularly when it is connected with cardiac problems. The drug has benefits in treating internal haemorrhage, epilepsy, inflammatory diseases and delirium tremens. Digitalis has a cumulative action whereby it is liable to accumulate in the body and then have poisonous effects. It should only be used under medical advice. Digitalis is an excellent antidote in ACONITE poisoning when given as a hypodermic injection.

Administered as: tincture, infusion, powdered leaves, solid extract, injection.

gale, sweet
Myrica gale

Common name: bayberry, English bog myrtle, Dutch myrtle, gale palustris.

Occurrence: a bushy shrub found in higher latitudes of the northern hemisphere; abundant in Scottish moors and bogs.

Parts used: the shrub.

Medicinal uses: aromatic, astringent. The leaves have been used as an emmenagogue and an abortifacient (induces abortion or miscarriage).

Administered as: dried leaves and infusion.

garlic *Allium sativum*

Common name: poor man's treacle.
Occurrence: cultivated throughout Europe since antiquity.
Parts used: the bulb.
Medicinal uses: antiseptic, diaphoretic, diuretic, expectorant,
stimulant. It may be externally applied as ointment, lotion,
antiseptic or as a poultice. Syrup of garlic is very good for
asthma, coughs, difficulty in breathing and chronic
bronchitis, while fresh juice has been used to ease tubercu-
lar consumption. The essential oil is commonly taken as a
supplement in the form of gelatine capsules. Several species
of wild garlic are used for both medicinal and dietary purposes.
Administered as: expressed juice, syrup, tincture, essential
oil, poultice, lotion and ointment.

golden rod *Solidago virgaurea*

Common name: verge d'or, solidago, goldruthe, woundwort,
Aaron's rod.
Occurrence: found wild in woods in Britain, Europe, Central
Asia and North America but also a common garden plant.
Parts used: the leaves contain tannin, with some bitter and
astringent chemicals that are unknown.
Medicinal uses: aromatic, stimulant, carminative. This herb is
astringent and diuretic and is highly effective in curing gravel
and urinary stones. It aids weak digestion, stops sickness
and is very good against diphtheria. As a warm infusion it is
a good diaphoretic drug and is used as such to help painful
menstruation and amenorrhoea (absence or stopping of
menstrual periods).
Administered as: fluid extract, infusion, spray.

hawthorn *Crataegus oxyacantha*

Common name: may, mayblossom, quickthorn, white-thorn,
haw, hazels, gazels, halves, hagthorn, ladies meat, bread
and cheese tree, maybush.

Occurrence: a familiar tree in Great Britain, Europe, North Africa and Western Asia.

Parts used: the dried fruits, which contain the chemical amyddalin.

Medicinal uses: cardiac, diuretic, astringent, tonic. Mainly used as a cardiac tonic in organic and functional heart problems, e.g. hypertrophy, dyspnoea, heart oppression. A decoction of the flowers and berries is good at curing sore throats, and is utilized as a diuretic in dropsy and kidney disorders.

Administered as: liquid extract, decoction.

heartease *Viola tricolor*

Common name: wild pansy, love-lies-bleeding, loving idol, call-me-to-you, three-faces-under-a-hood, godfathers and godmothers, pink-eyed-John, flower o'luce, Jack-jump-up-and-kiss-me.

Occurrence: abundant all over Great Britain, in cornfields, gardens, waste ground and hedge banks; also distributed through Arctic Europe, north Africa, Siberia and north India.

Parts used: the whole herb, fresh and dried. The active chemicals within the plant include violine, mucilage, resin, salicylic acid and sugar.

Medicinal uses: diaphoretic and diuretic. Formerly held in high regard as a remedy for epilepsy, asthma and catarrhal infections, it has been utilized in blood disorders and heart diseases while a decoction of the flowers was recommended for skin diseases. In America, they use heartease as an ointment or poultice in eczema, and it is taken internally for bronchitis. People on the continent have used *Viola tricolor* for its mucilaginous, demulcent and expectorant qualities.

Administered as: decoction, ointment, poultice and tincture.

hellebore, black *Helleborus niger*

Common name: Christe herbe, Christmas rose, melampodium.

Occurrence: native of the mountains in central and southern

Europe, Greece and Asia Minor; in Britain it is a garden plant.

Parts used: the rhizome and root. the plant has two glucosides within it, helleborin and helleborcin, both of which are powerful poisons.

Medicinal uses: the drug has drastic purgative, emmenagogue and anthelmintic properties, but is a violent narcotic. It is of value in treating nervous disorders, hysteria and melancholia and was previously used in dropsy and ammenorrhoea. Given externally, the fresh root is violently irritant. The drug must be administered with great care.

Administered as: fluid extract, tincture, solid extract, powdered root or decoction.

hemlock   *Conium maculatum*

Common name: herb Bennet, spotted conebane, musquash root, beaver poison, poison hemlock, poison parsley, spotted hemlock, vex, vecksies.

Occurrence: common in hedges, meadows, waste ground and stream banks throughout Europe and also found in temperate Asia and North Africa.

Parts used: the leaves, fruits and seeds. The most important constituent of hemlock leaves is the alkaloid coniine, which is poisonous, with a disagreeable odour. Other alkaloids in the plant include methyl-coniine, conhydrine, pseudo-conhydrine, ethyl piperidine.

Medicinal uses: sedative, antispasmodic, anodyne. The drug acts on the centres of motion and causes paralysis and so it is used to remedy undue nervous motor excitability, e.g. teething, cramp and muscle spasms of the larynx and gullet. When inhaled, it is said to be good in relieving coughs, bronchitis, whooping cough and asthma. The method of action of *Conium* means it is directly antagonistic to the effects of strychnine and hence it is used as an antidote to strychnine poisoning and similar poisons. Hemlock has to be administered with care as narcotic poisoning may result from internal application and overdoses induce paralysis, with loss of speech and depression of respiratory function leading to death. Antidotes to hemlock poisoning are tannic acid, stimulants, e.g. coffee, MUSTARD and castor oil.

Administered as: powdered leaves, fluid extract, tincture, expressed juice of the leaves and solid extract.

honeysuckle   *Lonicera caprifolium*

Common name: Dutch honeysuckle, goat's leaf, perfoliate honeysuckle.
Occurrence: grows freely in Europe, Great Britain and through the northern temperate zone.
Parts used: the dried flowers and leaves.
Medicinal uses: expectorant, laxative. A syrup made of the flowers is used for respiratory diseases and asthma. A decoction of the leaves is laxative and is also good against diseases of the liver and spleen, and in gargles.
Administered as: syrup, decoction.

hops   *Humulus lupulus*

Occurrence: a native British plant, found wild in hedges and woods from Yorkshire southward; an introduced species to Scotland but also found in most countries of the northern temperate zone.
Parts used: the flowers, which contain a volatile oil, two bitter principles—lupamaric acid, lupalinic acid and tannin.
Medicinal uses: tonic, nervine, diuretic, anodyne, aromatic. The volatile oil has sedative and soporific effects while the bitter principles are stomachic and tonic. Hops are used to promote the appetite and enhance sleep. An infusion is very effective in heart disease, fits, neuralgia, indigestion, jaundice, nervous disorders and stomach or liver problems. Hop juice is a blood cleanser and is effective in remedying calculus problems. Externally, hops are used with CAMOMILE heads as

an infusion to reduce painful swellings or inflammation and bruises. This combination may also be used as a poultice.
Administered as: an infusion, tincture, poultice, expressed juice or tea.

houseleek   *Sempervivum tectorum*
Common name: Jupiter's eye, Thor's beard, bullock's eye, sengreen, ayron, ayegreen.
Occurrence: native to central and southern Europe and the Greek islands but introduced to Britain many centuries ago.
Parts used: fresh leaves.
Medicinal uses: refrigerant, astringent, diuretic. The bruised fresh leaves or its expressed juice are often applied as a poultice to burns, scalds, bumps, scrofulous ulcers and general skin inflammation. The juice is a cure for warts and corns. In large doses, houseleek juice is emetic and purgative. The plant was supposed to guard where it grew against fire, lightning and sorcery, hence it was grown on house roofs.

ivy, ground   *Glechoma hederacea*
Common name: alehoof, Gill-go-over-the-ground, haymaids, tun-hoof, hedgemaids, coltsfoot, robin-run-in-the-hedge.
Occurrence: very common on hedges and waste ground all over Great Britain.
Parts used: the whole herb.
Medicinal uses: diuretic, astringent, tonic and gently stimulant. It is good in relieving kidney diseases and indigestion. The tea is useful in pectoral complaints and in weakness of the digestive organs. The juice, when sniffed up the nose, is said to cure a headache and can be administered externally to ease bruises and black eyes. It has antiscorbutic qualities.
Administered as: fluid extract, expressed juice and infusion.

Jacob's ladder   *Polemonicum coeruleum*
Common name: Greek valerian, charity.

Occurrence: found wild in ditches and streams across England and southern Scotland.
Parts used: the herb.
Medicinal uses: diaphoretic, astringent, alterative, expectorant. A useful drug in fevers and inflammatory diseases, pleurisy etc. It induces copious perspiration and eases coughs, colds, bronchial and lung complaints.
Administered as: an infusion.

juniper   *Juniperus communis*
Occurrence: a common shrub native to Great Britain and widely distributed through many parts of the world.
Parts used: the berry and leaves.
Medicinal uses: the oil from the ripe berries is stomachic, diuretic and carminative and is used to treat indigestion, flatulence and kidney and bladder diseases. Its main use is in dropsy and aiding other diuretic herbs to ease the condition.
Administered as: essential oil from berries, essential oil from wood, fluid extract, liquid extract, solid extract.

knotgrass   *Polyganum aviculare*
Common name: centinode, ninety-knot, nine-joints, allseed, bird's tongue, sparrow tongue, red robin, Armstrong, cowgrass, hogweed, pigrush, swynel grass, swine's grass.
Occurrence: native around the globe; abundant on arable land, waste ground and roadside verges.
Parts used: the whole herb.
Medicinal uses: astringent, diuretic, anthelmintic, vulnerary and styptic. An infusion of the herb was used in diarrhoea, bleeding haemorrhoids and all haemorrhages. As a diuretic, it was said to expel stones and also parasitic worms. The fresh juice stops nosebleeds, if squirted up the nose and applied to the temples. As an ointment, it heals sores very well.
Administered as: expressed juice, infusion, decoction and ointment.

larch   *Pinus larix*

Common name: *Larix europaea*, *Abies larix*, *Larix decidua*,
Laricus cortex, European larch, Venice turpentine.
Occurrence: indigenous to hilly regions of central Europe
but introduced into Britain in 1639.
Parts used: the inner bark, which contains tannic acid,
larixinic acid and turpentine.
Medicinal uses: stimulant, diuretic, astringent, balsamic and
expectorant. It is useful as an external application for eczema
and psoriasis but is mainly used as a stimulant expectorant
in chronic bronchitis, internal haemorrhage and cystitis. Larch
turpentine has also been suggested as an antidote in cyanide
or opium poisoning and has been used as a disinfectant.
Administered as: fluid extract or syrup.

lavender, English   *Lavandula vera*

Occurrence: indigenous to mountainous regions in the
western Mediterranean and cultivated extensively in France,
Italy, England and Norway.
Parts used: the flowers and the essential oil, which contains
linalool, linalyl acetate, cineol, pinene, limonene and tannin.
Medicinal uses: aromatic, carminative, stimulant, nervine. It
is mainly used as a flavouring agent for disagreeable odours
in ointments or syrups. The essential oil taken internally is
restorative and a tonic against faintness, heart palpitations,
giddiness and colic. It raises the spirits, promotes appetite
and dispels flatulence. Externally, the oil relieves toothache,
neuralgia, sprains and rheumatism. The oil is utilized widely
in aromatherapy, often to very beneficial effects.
Administered as: fluid extract, tincture, essential oil, spirit,
infusion, tea, poultice, distilled water.

lettuce, wild   *Lactuca virosa*

Common name: lachicarium, strong-scented lettuce, green
endive, lettuce opium, acrid lettuce, laitue vireuse.

Occurrence: western and southern Europe, including Britain.
Parts used: the leaves, dried milk juice. Lactuarium is obtained
by cutting the stem in sections and collecting the latex juice.
It turns reddish-brown in colour when dried.
Medicinal uses: anodyne, sedative, narcotic, mild diaphoretic,
diuretic. The drug resembles a weak opium, without opium's
tendency to upset the digestion. It is used to allay irritable
coughs and infrequently as a sedative and narcotic. It is also
used for dropsy, inducing sleep and easing colic.
Administered as: powder, tincture, fluid extract, syrup,
alcoholic extract.

liquorice   *Glycyrrbiza glabra*
Common name: licorice, lycorys, *Liquiriba officinalis*.
Occurrence: a shrub native to southeast Europe and southwest Asia and cultivated in the British Isles.
Parts used: the root. The chief compound in the root is glychr-
rhizin, with sugar, starch, gum, asparagus, tannin and resin.
Medicinal uses: demulcent, pectoral, emollient. A popular
and well-known remedy for coughs, consumption and chest
complaints. Liquorice extract is included in cough lozenges
and pastilles, with sedatives and expectorants. An infusion
of bruised root and FLAX (linseed) is good for irritable coughs,
sore throats and laryngitis. It is used to a greater extent as a
medicine in China and other eastern countries. The herb is
used by brewers to give colour to stout and is employed in
the manufacture of chewing or smoking tobacco.
Administered as: powdered root, fluid extract, infusion,
solid extract.

marigold   *Calendula officinalis*
Common name: *Caltha officinalis*, golds, ruddes, marg gowles,
oculus Christi, marygold, garden marigold, solis sponsa.
Occurrence: a native of southern Europe and a common
garden plant in Britain.

Parts used: the petals and herb. Only the deep orange-flowered variety is of medicinal use.

Medicinal uses: stimulant, diaphoretic. Mainly used as a local remedy. Taken internally, an infusion of the herb prevents pus formation and externally is good in cleaning chronic ulcers and varicose veins. Formerly considered to be of benefit as an aperient and detergent to clear visceral obstructions and jaundice. A marigold flower, when rubbed onto a bee or wasp sting, was known to relieve pain and reduce swelling, while a lotion from the flowers was good for inflamed and sore eyes. The expressed juice of the plant was used to clear headaches and remove warts.

Administered as: infusion, distilled water and lotion.

marjoram   *Origanum vulgare*

Occurrence: generally distributed over Asia, Europe and North Africa and also found freely in England.

Parts used: the herb and volatile oil.

Medicinal uses: the oil has stimulant, carminative, diaphoretic, mildly tonic and emmenagogue qualities. As a warm infusion, it is used to produce perspiration and bring out the spots of measles as well as giving relief from spasms, colic and dyspeptic pain. The oil has been used externally as a rubefacient and liniment, and on cotton wool placed next to an aching tooth it relieves the pain. The dried herb may be used as a hot poultice for swellings, rheumatism and colic, while an infusion of the fresh plant eases a nervous headache.

Administered as: essential oil, poultice and infusion.

marshmallow   *Althaea officinalis*

Common name: mallards, mauls, schloss tea, cheeses, mortification, root, guimauve.

Occurrence: a native of Europe, found in salt marshes, meadows, ditches and riverbanks; locally distributed in England and introduced to Scotland.

Parts used: leaves, root and flowers. Marshmallow contains starch, mucilage, pectin, oil, sugar, asparagin, glutinous matter and cellulose.

Medicinal uses: demulcent, emollient. Very useful in inflammation and irritation of the alimentary canal and the urinary and respiratory organs. A decoction of the root is effective against sprains, bruises and muscle aches. When boiled in milk or wine it relieves diseases of the chest, e.g. coughs, bronchitis or whooping cough, and eases the bowels after dysentery without astringent effects. It is frequently given as a syrup to infants and children.

Administered as: infusion, decoction, syrup, fluid extract.

meadowsweet   *Spiraea ulmaria*
Common name: meadsweet, dolloff, queen of the meadow, bridewort, lady of the meadow.
Occurrence: common in Britain in meadows or woods.
Parts used: the herb.
Medicinal uses: aromatic, astringent, diuretic, alterative. It is good against diarrhoea, stomach complaints and blood disorders. It is highly recommended for children's diarrhoea and dropsy and was used as a decoction in wine to reduce fevers. It makes a pleasant drink when infused and sweetened with honey. It is also included in many herb beers.
Administered as: infusion, decoction.

mistletoe   *Viscum album*
Common name: European mistletoe, bird-lime mistletoe, herbe de la Croix, mystyldene, lignum crucis.
Occurrence: an evergreen, true parasitic plant found on several tree species including fruit and oak trees; found throughout Europe and Britain except in Scotland, where it is very rare.
Parts used: the leaves and young twigs. They contain mucilage, sugar, fixed oil, tannin and viscin, the active part of the plant.

Medicinal uses: nervine, antispasmodic, tonic and narcotic. It is highly recommended for epilepsy and other convulsive disorders, along with stopping internal haemorrhage. It has also been used in delirium, hysteria, neuralgia, nervous debility, urinary disorders and many other complaints arising from a weakened state of the nervous system. The berries are taken to cure severe stitches in the side, and the plant produces a sticky substance called bird-lime, which is applied to ulcers and sores. Mistletoe is excellent for reducing blood pressure and has been indicated to be a successful cure for chronic arthritis and in treating malignant tumours in the body.

Administered as: tincture, powdered leaves, infusion, fluid extract.

mustard, black   *Brassica nigra, Siriapis nigra*
Common name: *Brassica sinapioides*
Occurrence: wild throughout Europe, south Siberia, Turkey and North Africa and cultivated in England, Italy, Germany and the Netherlands as a condiment.
Parts used: the seeds, which contain an acrid, volatile oil, an active principle, the glucoside sinigrin and the enzyme myrosin. When the seeds are crushed with water, these latter two chemicals come into contact and form oil of mustard.
Medicinal uses: irritant, stimulant, diuretic and emetic. Mainly used as a poultice to relieve acute local pain, e.g. pneumonia, bronchitis and other respiratory organ diseases. The herb draws blood to the skin surface, easing congestion of the organs, headaches, neuralgia and spasms. The oil of mustard is a powerful irritant and rubefacient when undiluted, but is very useful when dissolved in spirit for chilblains, rheumatism and colic. A hot infusion of the seed is a stimulating footbath and aids removal of colds or headaches. Mustard flour, when taken internally, can act as an

emetic, aperient and alterative herb and may also cure hiccups. It is also a very good antiseptic and sterilizing agent and deodorizer.

Administered as: poultice, infusion, essential oil, seed flour, leaves.

nettle   *Urtica dioica, Urtica urens*

Common name: common nettle, stinging nettle.
Occurrence: widely distributed throughout temperate Europe and Asia, Japan, South Africa and Australia.
Parts used: the whole herb, which contains formic acid, mucilage, mineral salts, ammonia and carbonic acid.
Medicinal uses: astringent, stimulating, diuretic, tonic. The herb is anti-asthmatic and the juice of the nettle will relieve bronchial and asthmatic troubles, as will the dried leaves when burnt and inhaled. The seeds are taken as an infusion or in wine to ease consumption or ague. Nettles are used widely as a food source and are made into puddings, tea, beer, juice and used as a vegetable. A hair tonic or lotion can also be made from the herb. In the Highlands of Scotland, they were chopped, added to egg white and applied to the temples as a cure for insomnia.
Administered as: expressed juice, infusion, decoction, seeds, dried herb, dietary item.

nightshade, black   *Solarum nignum*

Common name: garden nightshade, petty morel.
Occurrence: a common plant in south England, seen less frequently in northern England and Scotland.
Parts used: the whole plant, fresh leaves. Both contain the active principle solanine, which is found in variable quantities within the plant throughout the year.
Medicinal uses: the bruised fresh leaves are used external to the body to ease pain and reduce inflammation. Juice of the leaves has been used for ringworm, gout and earache and is

supposed to make a good gargle or mouthwash when mixed with vinegar. This species of plant is reputed to be very poisonous, narcotic and sudorific, so is only utilized in very small doses, under careful supervision.

Administered as: infusion, expressed juice and fresh leaves.

oak   *Quercus robur*
Common name: common oak, tanner's bark
Occurrence: a tree widely dispersed over Europe.
Parts used: the bark.
Medicinal uses: slightly tonic, strongly astringent, antiseptic. It is very good in chronic diarrhoea, dysentery as a decoction and used as a gargle for sore throats. May also be used as an injection for leucorrhoea and applied locally for piles and bleeding gums. Water distilled from the oak buds was said to be good on any kind of inflammation.
Administered as: fluid extract, infusion, tincture, injection.

oats   *Avena sativa*
Common name: groats, oatmeal.
Occurrence: distributed across Europe, Great Britain and USA.
Parts used: the seeds that are made up of starch, gluten, albumen and other proteins, sugar, gum oil and salts.
Medicinal uses: nervine, stimulant, antispasmodic, *Avena* forms a nutritious and easily digested food for convalescent patients and exhaustion after fevers. It can be made into a demulcent enema, or a good emollient poultice. Oat extract or tincture is useful as a nerve and uterine tonic.
Administered as: fluid extract, tincture, enema, dietary item.

parsley   *Carum petroselinum*
Common name: *Apium petroselinum*, *Petroselinum lativum*, petersylinge, persely, persele.
Occurrence: first cultivated in Britain in 1548, now completely naturalized through England and Scotland.

Parts used: the root, seeds and leaves. The root is slightly
aromatic and contains starch mucilage, sugar, volatile oil
and apiin. Parsley seeds contain more volatile oil, which
consists of terpenes and apiol, an allyl compound.
Medicinal uses: carminative, tonic, aperient, diuretic. A
strong decoction of the root is used in gravel, stone, kidney
congestion, jaundice and dropsy. Bruised parsley seeds used
to be given against plague and intermittent fevers, while the
external application of the leaves may help to dispel
tumours. A poultice of the leaves is effective against bites
and stings of poisonous insects.
Administered as: fluid extract, essential oil, infusion,
ointment and poultice.

peppermint   *Mentha piperita*
Common name: brandy mint, curled mint, balm mint.
Occurrence: found across Europe; introduced into Britain
and growing widely in damp places and waste ground.
Parts used: the herb and distilled oil. The plant contains
peppermint oil, which consists of menthol, menthyl acetate
and isovalerate, menthone, cineol, pinene and limonene.
The medicinal qualities are found in the alcoholic chemicals.
Medicinal uses: stimulant, antispasmodic, carminative,
stomachic, oil of peppermint is extensively used in medicine
and commerce. It is good in dyspepsia, flatulence, colic and
abdominal cramps. The oil allays sickness and nausea, is
used for cholera and diarrhoea but is normally used with
other medicines to disguise unpalatable tastes and effects.
Peppermint water is in most general use and is used to raise
body temperature and induce perspiration. Peppermint tea
can help ward off colds and influenza at an early stage, can
calm heart palpitations and is used to reduce the appetite.
Administered as: infusion, distilled water, spirit, essential oil
and fluid extract.

plantain, common   *Plantago major*

Common name: broad-leaved plantain, ripple grass,
waybread, snakeweed, cuckoo's bread, Englishman's foot,
white man's foot, waybroad.

Occurrence: a familiar weed all over Europe, Great Britain
and other parts of the world.

Parts used: the root, leaves and flowers.

Medicinal uses: refrigerant, diuretic, deobstruent, astringent,
cooling, alterative. The plant has been used in inflammation
of the skin, malignant ulcers, intermittent fever, applied to
sores and as a vulnerary. The fresh leaves can stop bleeding
of minor wounds, relieve the pain of insect stings, nettles,
burns and scalds.

Administered as: expressed juice, poultice, infusion, fresh
leaves, fluid extract, decoction, ointment.

poppy, white   *Papaver somniferum*

Common name: opium poppy, mawseed.

Occurrence: indigenous to Turkey and Asia, cultivated in
Europe, Great Britain, Persia, India and China for opium
production.

Parts used: the capsules and flowers. The white poppy
contains 21 different alkaloids of which morphine,
narcotine, codeine, codamine and thebaine are the most
important.

Medicinal uses: hypnotic, sedative, astringent, expectorant,
diaphoretic, antispasmodic, anodyne. The use of this drug
dates back to Greek and Roman times. It is the best possible
hypnotic and sedative drug, frequently used to relieve pain
and calm excitement. It has also been used in diarrhoea,
dysentery and some forms of cough. The tincture of opium
is commonly called laudanum, and when applied externally
with soap liniment it provides quick pain relief.

Administered as: syrup, tincture, decoction and poultice.

primrose *Primula vulgaris*

Occurrence: a common wild flower found in woods, hedgerows and pastures throughout Great Britain.

Parts used: the root and whole herb. Both contain a fragrant oil called primulin and the active principle saponin.

Medicinal uses: astringent, antispasmodic, vermifuge, emetic. It was formerly considered to be an important remedy in muscular rheumatism, paralysis and gout. A tincture of the whole plant has sedative effects and is used successfully in extreme sensitivity, restlessness and insomnia. Nervous headaches can be eased by treatment with an infusion of the root, while the powdered dry root serves as an emetic. An infusion of primrose flowers is excellent in nervous headaches and an ointment can be made out of the leaves to heal and salve wounds and cuts.

Administered as: infusion, tincture, powdered root and ointment.

quince *Cydonia oblongata*

Common name: quince seed, *Cydonica vulgaris*.

Occurrence: grown in England for its fruit but native to Persia.

Parts used: the fruit and seeds.

Medicinal uses: astringent, mucilaginous, demulcent. The fruit is used to prepare a syrup that is added to drinks when ill, as it restrains looseness of the bowels and helps relieve dysentery and diarrhoea. The soaked seeds form a mucilaginous mass similar to that produced by FLAX. A decoction of the seeds is used against gonorrhoea, thrush and in irritable conditions of the mucous membranes. The liquid is also used as a skin lotion or cream and administered in eye diseases as a soothing lotion.

Administered as: syrup, decoction or lotion.

ragwort *Senecio jacobaea*

Common name: St James's wort, stinking nanny,

staggerwort, ragweed, dog standard, cankerwort, stammerwort, fireweed.
Occurrence: an abundant wild plant, widely distributed over Great Britain, Europe, Siberia and northwest India.
Parts used: the herb.
Medicinal uses: diaphoretic, detergent, emollient, cooling, astringent. The leaves were used as emollient poultices, while the expressed juice of the herb was utilized as a wash in burns, eye inflammation, sores and cancerous ulcers. It has been successful in relieving rheumatism, sciatica, gout and in reducing inflammation and swelling of joints when applied as a poultice. Ragwort makes a good gargle for ulcerated throats and mouths and a decoction of its root is said to help internal bruising and wounds. The herb was previously thought to be able to prevent infection. This plant is poisonous to cattle and should be removed from their pastures. The alkaloids in the ragwort have cumulative effects in the cattle and low doses of the chemical eaten over a period of time can built up to a critical level, where the cattle show obvious symptoms and death then results. It is uncertain if sheep are also susceptible to this chemical.
Administered as: poultice, infusion and decoction.

rhubarb, English   *Rheum rhaponticum*
Common name: garden rhubarb, bastard rhubarb, sweet round-leaved dock, *Rheum officinale*.
Occurrence: cultivation started in England around 1777 and spread throughout Britain; it grows wild or near dwellings.
Parts used: the rhizome and root. The stem and leaves of the plant contain potassium oxalate in quantity and some people are more sensitive to these salts and should avoid eating the plant. People with gout or those subject to urinary irritation should avoid the plant as well.
Medicinal uses: stomachic, aperient, astringent, purgative.

This plant has a milder action than its relative, Turkey rhubarb (*Rheum palmatum*). It has a milder purgative effect and is particularly useful for stomach troubles in infants and looseness of the bowels. In large doses, rhubarb has a laxative effect. A decoction of the seed is proposed to ease stomach pain and increase the appetite. Rhubarb leaves were formerly used as a vegetable in the 19th century, and several fatal cases of poisoning were recorded.
Administered as: decoction and powdered root.

rosemary   *Rosmarinus officinalis*
Common name: Polar plant, compass-weed, compass plant, romero, *Rosmarinus coronarium*.
Occurrence: native to the dry hills of the Mediterranean, from Spain westward to Turkey; a common garden plant in Britain, cultivated prior to the Norman Conquest.
Parts used: the herb and root. Oil of rosemary is distilled from the plant tops and used medicinally. Rosemary contains tannic acid, a bitter principle, resin and a volatile oil.
Medicinal uses: tonic, astringent, diaphoretic, stimulant. The essential oil is also stomachic, nervine and carminative, and cures many types of headache. It is mainly applied externally as a hair lotion that is said to prevent baldness and dandruff. The oil is used externally as a rubefacient and is added to liniments for fragrance and stimulant properties. Rosemary tea can remove headache, colic, colds and nervous diseases and may also lift nervous depression.
Administered as: infusion, essential oil and lotion.

sage, common   *Salvia officinalis*
Common name: garden sage, red sage, sawge, broad-leaved white sage, *Salvia salvatrix*.
Occurrence: native to the northern Mediterranean and cultivated through Britain, France and Germany.
Parts used: the leaves, whole herb. The herb contains a

volatile oil, tannin and resin and is distilled to produce sage oil. This is made up of salvene, pinene, cineol, vorneol, thujone and some esters.

Medicinal uses: stimulant, astringent, tonic, carminative, aromatic. Sage makes an excellent gargle for relaxed throat and tonsils, bleeding gums, laryngitis and ulcerated throat. Sage tea is valuable against delirium of fevers, nervous excitement and accompanying brain and nervous diseases; as a stimulant tonic in stomach and nervous system complaints and in weak digestion. It also works as an emmenagogue, in treating typhoid fever, bilious and liver problems, kidney troubles and lung or stomach haemorrhages. The infusion is used in head colds, quinsy, measles, painful joints, lethargy, palsy and nervous headaches. Fresh leaves are rubbed on the teeth to cleanse them and strengthen gums—even today sage is included in toothpowders. The oil of sage was used to remove mucus collections from the respiratory organs and is included in embrocations for rheumatism. The herb is also applied warm as a poultice.

Administered as: infusion, essential oil, tea and poultice.

self-heal   *Prunella vulgaris*
Common name: prunella, all-heal, hook-heal, slough-heal, brunella, heart of the earth, blue curls, siclewort.
Occurrence: a very abundant wild plant in woods and fields all over Europe and Great Britain.
Parts used: the whole herb, containing a volatile oil, a bitter principle, tannin, sugar and cellulose.
Medicinal uses: astringent, styptic and tonic. An infusion of the herb is taken internally for sore throats, internal bleeding, leucorrhoea and as a general strengthener.
Administered as: infusion, injection and decoction.

snapdragon   *Antirrhinum magus*
Common name: calves snout, lyons snap.

Occurrence: naturalized in Great Britain as a garden plant.
Parts used: the leaves.
Medicinal uses: bitter, stimulant. The fresh leaves have been applied as a poultice to tumours an ulcers. In old herbals, it is mentioned that the herb protects against witchcraft and that it makes the wearer 'look gracious in the sight of people'.
Administered as: poultice.

sorrel   *Rumex acetosa*

Common name: garden sorrel, green sauce, sour grabs, sour suds, cuckoo sorrow, cuckoo's meate, gowke-meat.
Occurrence: indigenous to Britain and found in moist meadows throughout Europe.
Parts used: the leaves, dried and fresh.
Medicinal uses: refrigerant, diuretic, antiscorbutic. Sorrel is given as a cooling drink in all febrile conditions and can help correct scrofulous deposits. Its astringent qualities meant it was formerly used to stop haemorrhages and was applied as a poultice on cutaneous tumours. Sorrel juice and vinegar are said to cure ringworm, while a decoction was made to cure jaundice, ulcerated bowel, and gravel and stone in the kidneys.
Administered as: expressed juice, decoction, poultice and dried leaves.

St John's wort   *Hypericum perforatum*

Occurrence: found in woods, hedges, roadsides and meadows across Britain, Europe and Asia.
Parts used: the herb and flowers.
Medicinal uses: aromatic, astringent, resolvent, expectorant, diuretic and nervine. It is generally utilized in all pulmonary complaints, bladder trouble, suppression of urine, dysentery, diarrhoea and jaundice. It is good against hysteria, nervous depression, haemorrhages, coughing up blood and dispelling worms from the body. If children have a problem with

night incontinence, an infusion of St John's wort taken
before bed will stop the problem. The herb is used externally to break up hard tissues, e.g. tumours, swollen, hard
breasts when feeding young infants and bruising.
Administered as: an infusion and poultice.

strawberry
Fragaria vesca
Occurrence: found through the whole of the northern
hemisphere, excluding the tropics.
Parts used: the leaves, which contain cissotanic, malic and
citric acids, sugar, mucilage and a volatile aromatic chemical
that is, as yet, unidentified.
Medicinal uses: laxative, diuretic, astringent. The berries are
of great benefit for rheumatic gout while the root is good
against diarrhoea. The leaves have similar properties and are
used to stop dysentery. Fresh strawberries remove
discolouration of the teeth if the juice is left on for about
five minutes and then the teeth are cleaned with warm
water, to which a pinch of bicarbonate of soda has been
added. Sunburn could be relieved by rubbing a cut strawberry over a freshly washed face.
Administered as: infusion, fresh berries.

sundew
Drosera rotundifolia
Common name: round-leaved sundew, dew plant, red rot,
youthwort, rosa solis, herba rosellae, rosée du soleil.
Occurrence: an insectivorous plant found in bogs, wet
places and river edges throughout Britain, Europe, India,
China, North and South America and Russian Asia.
Parts used: the air-dried flowering plant.
Medicinal uses: pectoral, expectorant, demulcent, anti-
asthmatic. In small doses sundew is a specific in dry,
spasmodic, tickling coughs and is considered very good in
whooping cough, for which it may also be used as a
prophylactic drug. The fresh juice is used to remove corns

and warts. In America, the sundew has been advocated as a cure for old age and has been used with colloidal silicates in cases of thickening of arteries due to old age, or calcium or fat deposition.

Administered as: fluid extract, expressed juice, solid extract.

tansy   *Tanacetum vulgare*

Common name: buttons.

Occurrence: a hardy perennial plant, commonly seen in hedges and on waste ground all over Europe and Great Britain.

Parts used: the herb. It contains the chemicals tanacetin, tannic acid, a volatile oil, thujone, sugar and a colouring matter among others.

Medicinal uses: anthelmintic, tonic, emmenagogue, stimulant. Tansy is largely used for expelling worms from children. It is good in female disorders, like hysteria and nausea and in kidney weakness. The herb is also used for slight fevers, for allaying spasms and as a nervine drug. In large doses, the herb is violently irritant and induces venous congestion of the abdominal organs. In Scotland, an infusion was administered to cure gout. Tansy essential oil, when given in small doses, has helped in epilepsy and has also been used externally to help some eruptive diseases of the skin. Bruised fresh leaves can reduce swelling and relieve sprains, as can a hot infusion used as a poultice.

Administered as: essential oil, infusion, poultice, fresh leaves, solid extract.

thistle, holy   *Carbenia benedicta*

Common name: blessed thistle, *Cnicus benedictus, Carduus benedictus*.

Occurrence: a native of southern Europe and cultivated in Britain for hundreds of years.

Parts used: the whole herb which contains a volatile oil, a bitter crystalline compound, called cnicin, that is said to be similar to salicin in its properties.

Medicinal uses: tonic, stimulant, diaphoretic, emetic and emmenagogue. Useful as an infusion to weak and debilitating stomach conditions, creating appetite and preventing sickness. It is said to be good in all fevers, as a purifier of the blood and circulation and its main modern day use is for bringing on a proper supply of milk in nursing mothers. In large doses, however, holy thistle is a strong emetic, producing vomiting. It may be used as a vermifuge.

Administered as: infusion and fluid extract.

thyme   *Thymus vulgaris*

Common name: garden or common thyme, tomillo.

Occurrence: cultivated in most temperate countries in northern Europe.

Parts used: the herb. Thyme gives rise to oil of thyme after distillation of the fresh leaves. This oil contains the phenols, thymol and carvacrol, as well as cymene, pinene and borneol.

Medicinal uses: antiseptic, antispasmodic, tonic, carminative. The fresh herb, in syrup, forms a safe cure for whooping cough, as is an infusion of the dried herb. The infusion or tea is beneficial for catarrh, sore throat, wind spasms, colic and in allaying fevers and colds. Thyme is generally used in conjunction with other remedies in herbal medicine.

Administered as: fluid extract, essential oil and infusion.

valerian   *Valeriana officinalis*

Common name: all-heal, great wild valerian, amantilla, setwall, sete-wale, capon's tail.

Occurrence: found throughout Europe and northern Asia; common in England in marshy thickets, riverbanks and ditches.

Parts used: the root, which contains a volatile oil, two alkaloids called chatarine and valerianine as well as several unidentified compounds.

Medicinal uses: powerful nervine, stimulant, carminative anodyne and antispasmodic herb. It may be given in all cases of nervous debility and irritation as it is not narcotic. The expressed juice of the fresh root has been used as a narcotic in insomnia and as an anticonvulsant in epilepsy. The oil of valerian is of use against cholera and in strengthening eyesight. A herbal compound containing valerian was given to civilians during World War II to reduce the effects of stress caused by repeated air raids.

Administered as: fluid extract, tincture, essential oil, solid extract, expressed juice.

vervain   *Verbena officinalis*

Common name: herb of grace, herbe sacrée. herba veneris, *Verbena hastata*.

Occurrence: grows across Europe, China, Japan and North Africa; also found in England by roadsides and in sunny fields.

Parts used: the herb. Vervain contains a peculiar tannin, which has not yet been fully investigated.

Medicinal uses: nervine, tonic, emetic, sudorific, astringent, diaphoretic, antispasmodic. This herb is recommended in many complaints including intermittent fevers, ulcers, pleurisy, ophthalmic disorders and is said to be a good galactogogue. May also be administered as a poultice to ease headache, ear neuralgia, rheumatism and taken as a decoction to ease bowel pain during purging. Vervain is often applied externally for piles.

Administered as: fluid extract, decoction.

violet   *Viola adorata*

Common name: blue violet, sweet violet, sweet-scented violet.

Occurrence: native to Britain and found widely over Europe, northern Asia and North America.

Parts used: the dried flowers and leaves and whole plant when fresh.

Medicinal uses: antiseptic, expectorant, laxative. The herb is mainly taken as syrup of violets, which has been used to cure the ague, epilepsy, eye inflammation, pleurisy, jaundice and sleeplessness, which are some of the many other complaints that benefit from treatment with this herb. The flowers possess expectorant properties and have long been used to treat coughs. The flowers may also be crystallized as a sweetmeat or added to salads. The rhizome is strongly emetic and purgative and has violent effects when administered. The seeds also have purgative and diuretic effects and are beneficial in treating urinary complaints and gravel. In the early 20th century, violet preparations were used to great effect against cancer. Fresh violet leaves are made into an infusion that was drunk regularly, and a poultice of the leaves was applied to the affected area. The herb has been used successfully to both allay pain and perhaps cure the cancer. It is said to be particularly good against throat cancer.
Administered as: infusion, poultice, injection, ointment, syrup and powdered root.

walnut *Juglans nigra*
Common name: carya, Jupiter's nuts, *Juglans regia*.
Occurrence: cultivated throughout Europe and probably native to Persia.
Parts used: the bark and leaves. The active principle of the walnut tree is nucin or juglon, while the kernels also contain oil, mucilage, albumin, cellulose, mineral matter and water.
Medicinal uses: alterative, laxative, detergent, astringent. The bark and leaves are used in skin problems, e.g. scrofulous diseases, herpes, eczema and for healing indolent ulcers. A strong infusion of the powdered bark has purgative effects, while the walnut has various properties dependent upon its stage of ripeness. Green walnuts are anthelmintic and vermifuge in action and are pickled in vinegar, which is

then used as a gargle for sore and ulcerated throats. The wood is used for furniture, gun stocks and for cabinets. Walnut oil expressed from the kernels is used in wood polishing, painting and is used as butter or frying oil.
Administered as: fluid extract, infusion, expressed oil, whole fruit.

willow, white   *Salix alba*
Common name: European willow.
Occurrence: a large tree growing in moist places and running streams around Great Britain and Europe.
Parts used: the bark and leaves. The bark contains tannin and salicin.
Medicinal uses: tonic, antiperiodic, astringent. The bark has been used in febrile diseases of rheumatic or gouty origin, diarrhoea and dysentery. It has been used in dyspepsia connected with digestive organ disorders. The bark has also been of benefit in convalescence after acute diseases and against parasitic worms.
Administered as: decoction, powdered root.

witch hazel   *Hanamelis virginiana*
Common name: spotted alder, winterbloom, snapping hazelnut.
Occurrence: native to the USA and Canada.
Parts used: the dried bark, both fresh and dried leaves. The leaves contain tannic and gallic acids, volatile oil and an unknown bitter principle. The bark contains tannin, gallic acid, a physterol, resin, fat and other bitter and odorous bodies.
Medicinal uses: astringent, tonic, sedative. Valuable in stopping internal and external haemorrhages and in treating piles. Mainly used for bruises, swelling, inflammation and tumours as a poultice. It may also be utilized for diarrhoea, dysentery and mucous discharges. A decoction is used against tuberculosis, gonorrhoea, menorrhagia and the

debilitated state resulting from abortion. Tea made from the bark or leaves aids bleeding of the stomach, bowel complaints and may be given as an injection for bleeding piles. Witch hazel is used to treat varicose veins as a moist poultice, as an extract to ease burns, scalds and insect and mosquito bites, and to help inflammation of the eyelids.
Administered as: liquid extract, injection, tincture, lotion, ointment, suppositories, poultice, infusion and decoction.

woundwort *Stachys palustris*
Common name: all-heal, panay, opopanewort, clown's woundwort, rusticum vulna herba, downy woundwort, stinking marsh stachys.
Occurrence: common to marshy meadows, riversides and ditches in most parts of Great Britain.
Parts used: the herb.
Medicinal uses: antiseptic, antispasmodic. The herb relieves cramp, gout, painful joints and vertigo, while bruised leaves will stop bleeding and encourage healing when applied to a wound. Woundwort had an excellent reputation as a vulnerary among all of the early herbalists. A syrup made of the fresh juice will stop haemorrhages and dysentery when taken internally. The tuberous roots are edible as are the young shoot, which resemble asparagus.
Administered as: poultice or syrup.

Classification of Herbs by Action

alterative: anemone pulsatilla, bittersweet, blue flag, burdock, burr marigold, celandine, clover (red), dock (yellow), elder, Jacob's ladder, meadowsweet, plantain (common), walnut.
anodyne: aconite, camomile, hemlock, hops, lettuce (wild), poppy (white), valerian.
anthelmintic: aloes, hellebore (black), knotgrass, tansy, walnut.

antiperiodic: willow (white).

antiscorbutic: sorrel.

antiseptic: avens, costmary, garlic, oak, thyme, violet, woundwort.

antispasmodic: anemone pulsatilla, belladonna, camomile, clover (red) cowslip, daisy (ox-eye), hemlock, mistletoe, oats, peppermint, poppy (white), primrose, thyme, valerian, vervain, woundwort.

aperient: club moss, costmary, couchgrass, dandelion, elder, feverfew, parsley, rhubarb.

aphrodisiac: celery.

aromatic: avens, basil, birthwort, caraway, dill, fennel, gale (sweet), golden rod, hops, lavender, meadowsweet, sage (common), St John's wort.

astringent: alder, avens, birch, blackberry, comfrey, costmary, dog-rose, elder, elm, evening primrose, eyebright, gale (sweet), golden rod, hawthorn, houseleek, ivy (ground), Jacob's ladder, knotgrass, larch, meadowsweet, nettle, oak, plantain (common), poppy (white), primrose, quince, ragwort, rhubarb, rosemary, sage (common), self-heal, St John's wort, strawberry, vervain, walnut, willow (white), witch hazel.

balsamic: larch.

bitter: birch, feverfew, snapdragon.

cardiac: asparagus, butterbur, foxglove, hawthorn.

carminative: balm, basil, caraway, catmint, celery, dill, fennel, feverfew, golden rod, juniper, lavender, marjoram, parsley, peppermint, sage (common), thyme, valerian.

cathartic: blue flag, bogbean, broom, bryony (white).

cooling: basil, cucumber, plantain (common), ragwort, sorrel, witch hazel.

demulcent: chickweed, coltsfoot, comfrey, couchgrass, elm, flax, liquorice, marshmallow, quince, sundew.

deobstruent: bogbean, plantain (common).

59

detergent: blackcurrant, ragwort, walnut.

diaphoretic: aconite, anemone pulsatilla, balm, blackcurrant, boneset, burdock, burr marigold, catmint, elder, garlic, heartease, Jacob's ladder, lettuce (wild), marigold, marjoram, poppy (white), ragwort, rosemary, thistle (holy), vervain.

diuretic: arnica, asparagus, belladonna, bittersweet, blackcurrant, blue flag, broom, burdock, burr marigold, butterbur, celandine, celery, club moss, couchgrass, cucumber, daisy (ox-eye), dandelion, elder, elm, foxglove, garlic, golden rod, hawthorn, heartease, hops, houseleek, ivy (ground), juniper, knotgrass, larch, lettuce (wild), meadowsweet, mustard (black), nettle, parsley, plantain (common), sorrel, St John's wort, strawberry.

emetic: daffodil, elder, mustard (black), primrose, thistle (holy), vervain.

emmenagogue: aloes, catmint, feverfew, gale (sweet), hellebore (black), marjoram, tansy, thistle (holy).

emollient: cucumber, flax, liquorice, marshmallow, ragwort.

expectorant: boneset, coltsfoot, comfrey, elder, garlic, honeysuckle, Jacob's ladder, larch, poppy (white), St John's wort, sundew, violet.

febrifuge: aconite, avens, balm, blackcurrant, bogbean, boneset.

galactogogue: vervain.

hydrogogue: bryony (white).

hypnotic: poppy (white).

irritant: bryony (white), mustard (black).

laxative: asparagus, boneset, dock (yellow), elder, honeysuckle, strawberry, violet, walnut.

mydriatic: belladonna.

narcotic: belladonna, bittersweet, hellebore (black), lettuce (wild), mistletoe, nightshade (black).

nervine: anemone pulsatilla, celery, club moss, hops, lavender, mistletoe, oats, St John's wort, valerian, vervain.

nutritive: oats.

pectoral: dog-rose, flax, liquorice, sundew.

purgative: aloes, celandine, cucumber, elder, hellebore (black), rhubarb.

refrigerant: blackcurrant, catmint, chickweed, dog-rose, houseleek, plantain (common), sorrel.

resolvent: bittersweet, St John's wort.

sedative: aconite, asparagus, belladonna, clover (red), cowslip, evening primrose, foxglove, hemlock, lettuce (wild), poppy (white), witch hazel.

stimulant: arnica, birthwort, blue flag, boneset, butterbur, caraway, catmint, celery, dill, elder, fennel, feverfew, garlic, golden rod, ivy (ground), larch, lavender, marigold, marjoram, mustard (black), nettle, oats, peppermint, rosemary, sage (common), snapdragon, tansy, thistle (holy), valerian.

stomachic: avens, camomile, dill, fennel, juniper, peppermint, rhubarb.

styptic: avens, knotgrass, self-heal.

sudorific: avens, nightshade (black), vervain.

taenicide: cucumber.

tonic: alder, avens, blackberry, bogbean, boneset, butterbur, catmint, celery, camomile, coltsfoot, daisy (ox-eye), dandelion, dock (yellow), elm, eyebright, foxglove, hawthorn, hops, ivy (ground), marjoram, mistletoe, nettle, oak, parsley, rosemary, sage (common), self-heal, tansy, thistle (holy), thyme, vervain, willow (white), witch hazel.

vermifuge: aloes, primrose, walnut.

vulnerary: arnica, comfrey, knotgrass.

Medical Terms

alterative: a term given to a substance that speeds up the renewal of the tissues, so that they can carry out their functions more effectively.

anodyne: a drug that eases and soothes pain.

anthelmintic: a substance that causes the death or expulsion of parasitic worms.

antiperiodic: a drug that prevents the return of recurring diseases, e.g. malaria.

antiscorbutic: a substance that prevents scurvy and contains necessary vitamins, e.g. vitamin C.

antiseptic: a substance that prevents the growth of disease-causing micro-organisms, e.g. bacteria, without causing damage to living tissue. It is applied to wounds to cleanse them and prevent infection.

antispasmodic: a drug that diminishes muscle spasms.

aperient: a medicine that produces a natural movement of the bowel.

aphrodisiac: a compound that excites the sexual organs.

aromatic: a substance that has an aroma.

astringent: a substance that causes cells to contract by losing proteins from their surface. This causes localized contraction of blood vessels and tissues.

balsamic: a substance that contains resins and benzoic acid and that is used to alleviate colds and abrasions.

bitter: a drug that is bitter-tasting and is used to stimulate the appetite.

cardiac: compounds that have some effect on the heart.

carminative: a preparation to relieve flatulence and any resultant griping.

cathartic: a compound that produces an evacuation of the bowels.

cooling: a substance that reduces the temperature and cools the skin.

demulcent: a substance that soothes and protects the alimentary canal.

deobstruent: a compound that is said to clear obstructions, and open the natural passages of the body.

detergent: a substance that has a cleansing action, either internally or on the skin.

diaphoretic: a term given to drugs that promote perspiration.

diuretics: applied to substances that stimulate the kidneys and increase urine and solute production.

emetic: a drug that induces vomiting.

emmenagogue: a compound that is able to excite the menstrual discharge.

emollient: a substance that softens or soothes the skin.

expectorant: a group of drugs that are taken to help in the removal of secretions from the lungs, bronchi and trachea.

febrifuge: a substance that reduces fever.

galactogogue: an agent that stimulates the production of breast milk or increases milk flow.

hydrogogue: applied to substances that have the property of removing accumulations of water or serum.

hypnotic: drugs or substances that induce sleep.

irritant: a general term encompassing any agent that causes irritation of a tissue.

laxative: a substance that is taken to evacuate the bowel or soften stools.

mydriatic: a compound that causes dilation of the pupil.

nervine: a name given to drugs that are used to restore the nerves to their natural state.

narcotic: a drug that leads to a stupor and complete loss of awareness.

nutritive: compounds that are nourishing to the body.

pectoral: applied to drugs that are a remedy in treating chest and lung complaints.

purgative: the name given to drugs or other measures that produce evacuation of the bowels. This has normally a more severe effect than aperients or laxatives.

refrigerant: a substance that relieves thirst and produces a feeling of coolness.

resolvent: a substance that is applied to swellings to reduce them in size.

rubefacient: a compound that causes the skin to redden and peel off. Causes blisters and inflammation.

sedative: a drug that lessens tension, anxiety and soothes over-excitement of the nervous system.

stimulant: a drug or other agent that increases the activity of an organ or system within the body.

stomachic: name given to drugs that treat stomach disorders.

styptic: applications that check bleeding by blood vessel contraction or by causing rapid blood clotting.

sudorific: a drug or agent that produces copious perspiration.

taenicide: drugs that are used to expel tapeworms from the body.

tonic: substances that are traditionally thought to give strength and vigour to the body and that are said to produce a feeling of well-being.

vermifuge: a substance that kills, or expels, worms from the intestines.

vulnerary: a drug that is said to be good at healing wounds.